Healthy Leadership in Healthcare

The Pope Francis Formula

Erny Gillen

translated by Johanna Ellsworth

edited by Lesley-Anne Knight and Mark Newman

Moral Factory S.à.r.l
71, rue due Viaduc
Esch-sur-Alzette
Grand-Duchy of Luxembourg
office@moralfactory.com

Cover by Kirsten Lenz
© Photo: Lex Kleren, LW

First English Edition 2016

Copyright © 2016 Erny Gillen

All rights reserved.

ISBN-10: 1536843865
ISBN-13: 978-1536843866

The Pope Francis Leadership Formula deserves not only admiration but also courageous application around the world. Through this publication, I hope to contribute towards its general understanding and praxis – and not only in the field of healthcare!

CONTENTS

Acknowledgments	i
Foreword	1
Introduction	6
PART I: FOUR CASE STUDIES	
I – 1 Starting point and diagnosis	11
I – 2 The Leadership Formula	15
I – 3 The sick take their lives in hand	18
I – 4 How healthcare professionals lead the relationship with patients	26
I – 5 The physician-patient conversation as a special leadership challenge	36
I – 6 The leadership formula in hospital management	43
I – 7 Use and benefits of the formula	50
PART II: LEADERSHIP TOWARDS AN OPEN FUTURE	
II – 1 The way forward	55
II – 2 The Pope Francis Leadership Formula	60
II – 3 Why time is worth more than space to ethical leaders	63
II – 4 Why unity is worth more than conflict to ethical leaders	69
II – 5 Why realities are worth more than ideas to ethical leaders	73
II – 6 Why the whole is worth more than the part to ethical leaders	77
Conclusion	81
About the author	84

ACKNOWLEDGMENTS

With deep gratitude for the ministry he offers to the world and the Catholic Church, I dedicate this booklet to Pope Francis, an inspirational leader who shares his Formula with all.

I am both humbled and encouraged by the Foreword contributed by Oscar Andrés Cardinal Rodríguez Maradiaga S.D.B. who has made such a great personal contribution to the mission Pope Francis took on when he was elected.

I was motivated to produce an English edition of *Healthy Leadership in Healthcare* by colleagues and scholars I met during my sabbatical in Boston, where Ethics and Leadership became established as the core of my current professional venture. I am grateful to Johanna Ellsworth for the English translation. I must also express my gratitude and deep respect for the work of my editors Mark Newman and Lesley-Anne Knight, whose thoughtful contributions and improvements have made this edition a truly new read for the English speaking community.

FOREWORD

BY OSCAR ANDRÉS CARDINAL RODRÍGUEZ
MARADIAGA, S.D.B.

Pope Francis walks his road without fear because he is carried and driven by his mission. Witnessing his emblematic actions and his inspiring words of wisdom and faith, it is not immediately obvious however that he is also a man who is a strong believer in method! During many years as a pastor, he developed not only a personal and incisive style but also a special method of orientation. With this powerful method and his deep relationship with God, he brings life and joy to our Church and to our world so that they can be re-energised in that same spirit. Neither our Church nor our world can accept standstill while people are suffering and in need, and while injustice and poverty prevail.

Almost daily we can watch and experience how his method brings movement to the new and the old. I am delighted to write this foreword for "Healthy Leadership in Healthcare. The Pope Francis Formula", in which Erny Gillen demonstrates that many people can benefit from the practical application of this formula. Using compelling case-studies, he shows how "The Pope Francis Method" can be applied in the realms of sickness and suffering to transform paralysed and blocked situations in a healthy way. He deals with patients' struggle for healing and opens hopeful avenues for them to courageously take their lives in hand, especially in the most critical moments.

As a former Professor of theological ethics, Erny Gillen pedagogically develops Pope Francis's Method using the image of an eight-sided dice (an octahedron) that helps us to understand and practise the Formula. The eight faces of this special dice present eight fields for action and reflection that we can influence and transform. Even as patients, we can take action and change our lives responsibly. He applies four priority preferences offered by the Holy Father, giving examples for patients, and also for doctors and nurses. As an expert in healthcare, who knows about the daily pain and needs of patients, he also demonstrates how the method can be applied to patient-doctor dialogue and to the governance and management of healthcare facilities.

A good method of orientation is especially valuable when the road is dangerous and the way ahead is obscured by fog and darkness. As a pastor, Pope Francis knows these situations because he has accompanied many, many people during his long and varied ministries. Today, he accompanies the worldwide Church and all women and men. Through his writings as Pope, he has offered us his special Method for our own orientation and leadership. In Part Two of his book, Erny Gillen shows how the Holy Father uses this method with wisdom to move ahead with reform of the Curia, and with the big questions concerning the family and, most importantly, our common home. With each step he encourages us not to halt, but to focus on the future and the common good. God walks the road with us and he comes to meet us from the future again and again. Time is God's messenger, Pope Francis tirelessly repeats, quoting blessed Petrus Faber.

As patients, doctors, nurses, pastors, social workers, managers and leaders of hospitals take up this book, I wish them courage as they study the underlying themes of methodic self-leadership and the leadership of people. As this method demonstrates, we all benefit when we understand why time is greater than space when we act, why unity prevails over conflicts, why realities are more important than ideas and finally why the whole is greater than the part. These four principles of the Holy Father may seem self-evident to some but will intrigue others as Erny Gillen patiently explains their application in healthcare and sheds light on their theological and ethical background.

In the long history of medicine doctors have always sought new methods to better cope with sickness. They extended their ears with stethoscopes and their eyes with echographs, X-ray or tomography to look deeper into the patient. Medical science has continually developed new medications and methods to improve health and enable patients to cope with illnesses. The art of medicine deserves our respect and admiration. This progress, together with good nursing and modern hospitals, creates refuges of humanity in which hurt and needy people find healing and care.

But hospitals can also be frightening places. When people are diagnosed with a serious illness, they face great uncertainty about what will happen. Afflicted and fragile patients are confronted with a mass of information, data and professionals, each addressing the issues in their particular expert language. Patients sometimes feel overwhelmed and dumbstruck. Yet, in the fog of this uncertainty, they are required to take risky and critical decisions about their lives and future. In such tough situations, where moral strength and personal leadership is necessary, The Pope Francis Method shows its full potential. It reduces complexity and offers guidance and orientation for all. At the same time, this method does not presuppose belief in God or a particular moral code. It is adaptable to the outlook of those using it. As a good method it has no hidden agenda and is not biased with regard to a predetermined outcome. It is an open method.

I would be delighted to see many Catholic and Christian healthcare facilities using this formula for the benefit of patients. But it can also be used by non-denominational facilities or corporations and become part of their endeavour of humanisation. Erny Gillen has produced a practical guide and syllabus, translating Pope Francis's concern into the situation of sick people and hospitals. He invites us to start and re-start again and again, to accept reality and to count on the mercy of God – a God who entrusts the power of life to our responsible hands. Protecting and preserving life also means being committed with our hearts and minds to humane healthcare systems from which no one is excluded.

Pope Francis has not kept his successful method to

himself, but made it available for all. Erny Gillen helps us to understand this method through the lens of a hospital, providing practical instruction and helpful hints on how it can positively transform a healthcare facility. With an innovative language-game, he supports a new type of dialogue in hospitals and thus lays the foundations for a specific corporate culture that is at the service of the sick on their road to recovery.

> Oscar Andrés Cardinal Rodríguez Maradiaga, S.D.B.
> Archbishop of Tegucigalpa, Honduras.

On the Solemnity of Christ the King, November 20th, 2016.

INTRODUCTION

Illness may sometimes result from leading an unhealthy lifestyle. But even a person being led through a spell of hospital treatment, may not always emerge in good health. The concepts of "health" and "leadership" have a profound inner connection in the life of every person, and in hospital this is particularly evident in the individual stories of patients, and in the healing processes that take place there. The hospital, as a modern refuge of humanity, leads people on a journey towards recovery, but the path is narrow and requires conscious ethical leadership that links everyone together in the service of health. This book therefore addresses patients as well as medical staff and introduces an innovative language-game both for self-leadership and guided leadership on the often arduous and precarious path of health.

Healthy Leadership also addresses those responsible for

the governance and management of hospitals. They create the environment and atmosphere necessary for the leadership of physicians, nurses, and patients, so it is even more important for them to have access to and to master the same language-game so that they may fulfil their specific responsibilities in the discourse about the hospital and its functions. Good organisation and synchronised language codes are essential for the whole facility. They enable everyone, in the true spirit of ethical leadership, to act responsibly at all levels.

Healthy Leadership, however, presents a moral argument that makes sense far beyond the hospital. The book thus also serves readers for whom "disease" could be replaced with "life crisis" and "hospital" with "counselling and support" services. If, for instance, you have lost your job, suffered bereavement or are encountering relationship problems, you can easily apply many aspects of *Healthy Leadership* to your current situation. Anyone who has reached a crossroads in their life, and does not know which way to turn, can use this book to regain their equilibrium and move forward.

Healthy Leadership has been inspired by the works of Pope Francis. His leadership is marked by humility and resolve on the one hand, and a clear, if less visible method, on the other. From the start, he has applied this method to help him and everyone else – independently from their belief systems – to make headway in difficult situations. At the same time, he has faith in those who have problems, or who create them, just as much as he has faith in an open future. His leadership approach is described in detail in his programmatic apostolic exhortation *Evangelii Gaudium* (The Joy of the Gospel).

In this book I have condensed Pope Francis' early Christian approach and his leadership principles (the results of which remain open) into a compact Leadership Formula so that as many people as possible may feel inspired by this method. The global effectiveness of these principles can be witnessed in the life and work of this Pope every day.

The first part of the book presents the Leadership Formula, using the example of sickness and hospital. From my experience in teaching and research in the fields of ethics and healthcare, I know the critical role diseases and hospitals play in any person's life. Nobody can escape the drastic changes sickness and suffering cause. In such a situation, a hospital can be experienced either as a refuge of humanity, or as a medical fortress in which patients (some of whom are also running away from themselves) subject themselves to the laws and logic of a strange host of gods clad in white. The leadership method of the Pope contrasts such simplifications and this "good-or-evil" approach with other polarities and balances that are often overlooked, although they can be found everywhere. He refers to eight coordinates that are interconnected in order to create a semantic and pragmatic field that allows for new types of movement. Part One of this book features four case studies and unfolds according to his formula, showing how it can help patients as much as physicians and nurses. I describe how it may serve the hospital management in guiding individuals and departments when approaching ethically complex issues, taking important executive decisions or making decision processes more transparent.

Part Two may be read independently of Part One. Some readers may find it worthwhile to read this fundamental part first. It shows how the formula has developed in the Pope's works and actions. It is a theological-ethical analysis that explains the system behind the work of this pope.

The Leadership Formula of Pope Francis is explicitly embedded in the social teachings of the Catholic Church and is situated at the interface between the Church and the world. Thus, it is dependent neither on faith nor religious denomination. Rather, it builds on the personal morals and resources of individuals who apply it, providing them with a method guided by reason that enables them to take action.

Many people are painfully aware that their good intentions do not produce results in their lives, because they fail to realise them. Moral demands on oneself will remain fruitless as long as individuals fail to lead their own lives or take their lives into their own hands. This experience of human inertia is mirrored in the wider worlds of business, religion and politics and can be seen in commercial corporations and religious organisations. Part Two focuses on how Pope Francis manages wisely and methodically to shake up the rigid structures of the Church and world politics, as demonstrated by his interventions for the World Climate Summit in Paris, and on Cuban-American relations, as well as his invitation to Israeli and Palestinian leaders to the Vatican Gardens.

I hope that you will make sound decisions on your way to developing your own leadership; may this book serve as a good personal guide for the road whenever you seek leadership yourself. Ethical leadership is an art you can learn and practise. Pope Francis is a shining example of how healthy leading can be accomplished. He is a follower of Jesus in the truest sense and I thank him with all my heart for his courage, and his Leadership Formula!

PART ONE

FOUR CASE STUDIES

I – 1: STARTING POINT AND DIAGNOSIS

Sickness and sorrow lead individuals, and societies, to unexpected crossroads in their lives – points at which decisions have to be made about the way forward. Sickness and sorrow can drive us to extraordinary achievements, but should we allow ourselves to be driven by them? Or should we practise independent and morally responsible leadership? The fearful question "Where do we go from here?" will accompany us throughout the first part of this book.

A considerable part of our ultramodern world and culture owes its existence to our efforts to safeguard and increase human health and happiness. But when danger threatens, how we react to it has a significant impact on our future. If we succumb to it too soon, we may miss out on the opportunity for a new chapter in our life. But if we persist in fighting blindly on, we may lose control of the situation – and of ourselves. When we cling to the familiar, we remain eternally in the present, without a past or a future. Of all our social achievements, the institution of the hospital represents, more than any other, a place where the lives, health and future of humans are at stake.

Where sickness or sorrow requires an answer, the two components and competencies expressed in "ethical leadership" are needed: firstly, a moral answer that shows the direction; and, secondly, a form of leadership that enables people to translate that answer into action. Morality without leadership is a theory for life within an Ivory Tower. And leadership without morality can quickly turn into frenetic activism without any orientation — and not only in hospitals.

As an ethicist and theologian, over the past 30 years I have focused intensely on moral dilemmas in the health system, in practice and in theory. As President of Caritas in Luxembourg and in Europe, I was able to experience and sometimes even contribute to developments in the Church and in society at the global level. Life has taught me to understand and acknowledge that radical personal decisions are extremely hard to make, and that taking them forward requires the courage to let go of old things and make room for the new.

The key ingredients for this book are four short sentences found in the writings of Pope Francis that obviously guide him as a leader, and make him an attractive role model far beyond the Catholic Church. These interconnected principles use four bipolar tensions to initiate movement. This is particularly important when there is a standstill — a clear indication that dying processes are under way and that life may be coming to an end.

Pope Francis applies his formula to influence world

politics when it concerns our common home, as well as the Church, for instance when he wants to encourage compassion in issues of marriage and family. I have asked myself if his method could be applied in different settings that require leadership in a new era and have come to the conclusion — as I hope this book shows — that it definitely can.

What can those people responsible for managing clinics and hospitals learn from this pope? What can sick people, their doctors, and nurses gain from his formula? Pope Francis is a political and religious leader who is accepted worldwide. For a long time, he has been leading and accompanying people making crucial decisions. He knows that, like a midwife, he must help new life come into this world.

Pope Francis has worked hard to develop competency as a leader[1] in his complicated life, not only as a Jesuit, master of novices and head of a province, but also as an exile and bishop of the poor. Today he can draw just as much on his wealth of personal and professional experience as on his vast education and training. As a man of the Church, he is aware of the importance of well-organised interaction between personal piety, sense of community, and a legally standardised public practice.

The concept applied by him — that I have summarised as the "Pope Francis Leadership Formula" — can be found in his guiding documents[1] and observed in his actions. Those who know his formula grasp his kind of leadership and its effectiveness better and more quickly. It describes the reality of his leadership and provides, in short form, extraordinarily lucid guidance for all leaders who want to try it. Francis carefully balances the powers

---

1) See Part Two of this book.

available to him to develop his leadership towards an open future in accordance with his purpose.

If leadership means moving purposefully in a certain direction, Pope Francis' method can be applied to one's individual health situation, the range of diagnostic and therapeutic treatments available, the decision-making processes between physicians and patients, as well as the management of health facilities. This is not a "magic formula" for all problems, but the Leadership Formula as a method helps to get decision-making situations that are stuck or rigid moving again. It triggers movement by gently changing existing balances. Old balances make room for new ones without making the whole structure collapse. It is clearly a "formula for the road".

Sickness is a common crisis in people's lives. It changes your balance and, whether you are wringing your hands or swallowing pills, it will force you to work out a new balance. The hard task for patients is first and foremost to take on the leadership and control of their own bodies. In this process they are assisted by doctors and nurses, with modern hospitals providing the framework.

I – 2: THE LEADERSHIP FORMULA

These are the key elements of the Pope Francis Leadership Formula:

Time is greater than space (EG 221)

Unity prevails over conflict (EG 226)

Realities are more important than ideas (EG 231)

The whole is greater than the part (EG 234)

The formula connects these four bipolar tensions that can be graphically represented as the opposing faces of an octahedron, like a special kind of eight-sided dice. A system of coordinates is created that stimulates movement. Where there was previously stasis and resignation, a new playing field is established, in which action becomes possible again.

My thesis is that, by creating a common coordinate system and introducing a method of dialogue, a common language can be established in hospitals, using the formula as an open didactic instrument. This novel language-game translates patients' questions and answers, as well as those of physicians and nurses, into a clear system that makes possible not only trans-professional communication, but also intrapersonal and interpersonal communication.

I will show how the Pope's leadership concept helps the sick and suffering to overcome their lethargy and despondency, while protecting them from unrealistic and unattainable dreams. It provides physicians with an instrument that enables them to apply their expertise and experience professionally as leaders, for the benefit of their patients. In doctor-patient dialogue, the leadership method develops its full potential, especially if physicians accept their role and responsibility as the patient's leader. Hospital managements can also use the formula to facilitate the continuous transparent development of their purpose.

When the purpose of an endeavour is unclear, ambiguous, or even non-existent, a leadership vacuum is created. This is less common in the health system, however, where there is an urgent imperative to improve and maintain patients' health. Working towards this clear purpose, the Leadership Formula can unfold its full power by addressing open or unasked questions. Its success is based on the moral strength of those working with the special dice and the formula it represents.

This part of the book is structured around the actors involved: the patient, the physician, the two of them in dialogue together, and the hospital management. Regarding the patient, a chronic disease will serve as an example; with the physician, it will be the intrapersonal dealing with death; for the doctor-patient conversation, it will be the decision-finding process; and regarding the hospital management, it will be the issue of how to limit costs.

This thematic approach shows how the Pope Francis Leadership Formula works in concrete situations, and lays the groundwork for the conclusion that difficult conversations about disease and hospitals can be conducted sensibly and reasonably. As good as it may be, a method cannot provide the content of the conversations or the moral points of view taken; but it can support and provide a common framework for understanding and communication. The eight-sided dice opens up a particular language-game that has health and healing at its centre. It marks out the field upon which the crucial question to be tackled is "Where do we go from here?"

I – 3: THE SICK TAKE THEIR LIVES IN HAND

For many people, illness starts with a persistent pain like a toothache. Or there is an unusual limitation to a familiar pattern of movements. Maybe the digestive system no longer works as it should. Suddenly, everything has changed, from one minute to the next. Your body feels different. Before the pain, you never had to think how to move or to chew, but now the habitual process is disrupted. Your first reaction may be to wait and see if the sensation goes away by itself. A harmless illness can quickly be passed by, without the need for further treatment or reflection, and you may be left with nothing more than an indelible memory of a traumatic experience.

However, to examine how the Leadership Method can be applied in practice, we will study the example of a chronic disease – in this case, a serious cardiovascular disorder. The experience of a minor heart attack illustrates how a person becomes slowly aware of their illness. If you have a heart attack and wake up in hospital, your sense of **space** and **time** changes abruptly. Even a glance at the big clock on the wall cannot tell you with certainty if it is day or night; you don't know whether you have been unconscious for hours, or for days. Furthermore, space has changed as abruptly as time – starting with the bed in which you find yourself, with tubes attached to you and strange sounds all around you. Your most intimate space — your body — feels different. There are unfamiliar sensations of tension and pressure. And you can feel your heart beating, which you hardly ever used to notice before.

The patient in a hospital bed, and later at home, will find that their time and space are no longer the same as before. However, the external environment keeps on functioning in the familiar space-time rhythms and coordinates. Spatially and temporally, the patient feels like they have fallen out of the old world, and it will require effort and work to synchronise the spaces and times of the lost world with those in the world that lies ahead. The continuity of life is broken, or at least interrupted. Patients have to re-define their time and space, for themselves and others.

Simple illnesses or minor injuries are obviously unlikely to trigger such life crises. Patients will just see the temporary interruption to their time-flow as a 'blip' in their systems and quickly return to their former coordinates. It is a disruption to life, but not a threat to life.

Chronically sick patients, however, are less able to ignore their spatial and temporal limitations; they will be constantly reminded of them. Serious disease makes strong demands on one's consciousness, and memories of times and spaces render the burden even heavier, since they seem irrevocably lost. In such a situation it helps to adjust the balance between the two poles of time and space towards time. Time can be re-shaped more quickly than the new space, which will take time to modify. What can be achieved through a quiet rest and a good sleep can sometimes come close to a miracle. But dealing with time during patients' waking hours, makes clear to their consciousness that time moves on and remains re-shapeable — even independently of the new spatial limitations of the body. Good ministers and smart visitors know what the gift of a book or music can mean to sick people. Patients can regain control over their own time again — just by reading a few lines or listening to music they have selected themselves. They are no longer just patients, and their illness no longer defines their whole life. They start to control their own time again, thus changing their space from the inside.

Giving time priority over physical space also changes the perception of the body. Time is simply more powerful than space. And so patients learn to "deal" with time so that it becomes impossible for the sick body to take up the whole space. Instead, it is assigned its new place and space in the patient's time. Concentrating only on the body is just as unhelpful as ignoring its needs. Patients can end their helplessness in the disease better if they give more weight to time than to space. When space is no longer everything and they have regained control over their changed time, they have the freedom to turn to the next area of tension in the octahedron: **conflicts** and **unity**.

What are the inner and bodily conflicts that can shatter the wholeness of a person who is chronically ill? Firstly, let's examine **inner conflicts**. Above all, these conflicts arise from the "self-portrait" patients have drawn and lived prior to the onset of their illness. If the patient suffering a heart attack is a senior manager, their identity as an invincible, indispensable person will shatter as soon as they find themselves in hospital. They will not enjoy being seen in their pyjamas by visiting colleagues or their chief executive. An athlete who suffers a heart attack will have to come to terms with the possible end of their career. An elderly retiree will start to grasp that they won't be taking part in the next hiking tour in the mountains. "Re-shaping" time can help in situations like these to disarm the conflict. But what realistic new self-portrait should the patient sketch out that they can further develop? Patients have to re-design their role in the realms of profession, leisure time, and family. If, for instance, their profession was their primary source of self-fulfilment, this crisis may well result in them spending more time at home with their family. If the heart attack was partly self-inflicted, because the patient had lost a sense of unity and thought they could lead three separate lives simultaneously, their laboured breathing will remind them that they have only one life.

The Leadership Formula of Pope Francis brings movement to the tension between **conflict** and **unity** by giving more weight to unity than to threatening conflicts. The Pope suggests that we should not avoid conflicts, but neither should we become too embroiled in them. He believes that the concerns involved in the most serious conflicts must be addressed. He seeks a solution in a new synthesis or a reconciliation of differences, but not in a struggle in which one argument is suppressed by another. Any true conflict merits attention and addresses an issue that needs to be resolved at a higher level. Pope Francis' formula may benefit patients' personal integrity and unity and help them to consider another kind of life as an alternative to the one that has just been disrupted. Looking for a solution to a conflict at a higher level is not about ignoring the legitimate issues of old conflicts. On the contrary: the issues that led to the inner conflicts in the first place should be integrated into the outline of the individual's new life. The aim is not to become a new person separated from one's old life and inner conflicts. People who deal with themselves and their inner conflicts in a new and different way will continue to be the same person, while changing the spaces and conditions they can effectively influence. With time, their continuity as an individual will become more apparent. They will accept themselves in this new existence and start living out of their newly built unity.

The same applies to the **bodily conflicts** that can accompany any chronic cardiovascular disease. Often this is about the conscious processes of moving and eating. Both have to do with human needs and familiar patterns of behaviour. Here it also helps to stay focused on unity, and not to get overly involved in a particular conflict regarding "movement" or "eating" or "relaxation". The unity — here in the sense of the patient's overall wellbeing — is more important than the individual conflict or the whole collection of conflicts. A new feeling for life and a new lifestyle do not come overnight; here, too, the first part of the formula, concerning time, is significant. The desirable bodily changes concern the whole person who wants to change, and not just some areas of conflict. If, for instance, an individual who does not like to swim steps into the pool each day, they will in time become a changed person who has re-invented themselves in a new daily rhythm — and will also have met new people and expanded their social environment in the process.

The next bipolar tension found in the Leadership Formula is that between **realities** and **ideas**. This is about "trial and error". The new self-portrait starts out as an idea about how you want to be in the future: more athletic, slimmer, more flexible, more relaxed, etc. Since realities are stronger than ideas, it is worth acknowledging that they take priority. This is what Pope Francis advocates in the third part of his Leadership Formula.

You cannot control your own life if you are no longer grounded and have lost your sense of reality. A surprising number of heart attacks are the result of an obsessive attraction to a self-portrait that does not reflect the reality of the body. The same danger exists with the new self-portrait that will be developed by patients after leaving hospital. They, too, may focus more on an "idea" about themselves than on their reality with its physical, mental, and spiritual limitations. No convalescent patient should recklessly evade this reality test.

The third part of the Leadership Formula ("Realities are more important than ideas") gives patients a simple method to test their ideas: If just one fact of reality disproves an idea, it is false. Thus, if recuperating patients cling to the idea of hiking again in three weeks' time and then feel sharp pains and shortness of breath when climbing stairs, the idea is probably false. They will do well to take a more realistic view of their situation and to align their ideas with their current reality.

The fourth bipolar tension (between the **whole** and the **part**) may bring clarity to the patient who is looking for a new orientation and self-portrait. The Pope's formula gives priority to the whole over the part. This can serve as a compass for patients who still feel lost in their new existence and need help with decisions. Their chronic illness has already changed them and their whole life. Their life must be reassembled according to a new "blueprint". Developing the image of the polyhedron used by Pope Francis, it is helpful to think of those self-supporting structures known in architecture, mathematics and art as tensegrity structures. These can be simple or highly complex shapes whose structure hangs in a flexible state of balance. They playfully demonstrate that an interconnected structure can be adjusted in multiple ways, so long as all the parts are moved simultaneously, which is the only way to prevent the structure from collapsing. Many patients find it helpful to think of their self-supporting bodies as a living tensegrity structure. What the interconnected skeleton and tendons clearly show also applies to those less visible elements of the body that are, for instance, permanently balancing glucose levels in the blood.

This imagery shows that overall balance is as important, or more important, than individual, injured parts. Focusing on wounds or fractures is less helpful than concentrating on a goal. After all, optimal balance is not achieved by staring at one's feet but rather by looking straight ahead. It is not the feet that are walking but rather the person who sets out to walk.

The four bipolar areas of tension of Pope Francis' leadership concept show dramatically the importance of steering these tensions (between time and space, unity and conflict, realities and ideas, and the whole and the part) in the right direction in order to move forward. This is particularly true in a crisis – a situation in which decisions need to be made.

Nevertheless, many patients dealing with illness will spontaneously choose the opposite pole because they believe this will provide the solution to their ailment. They will focus all their attention on the space, the conflict, ideas, or a part of themselves, as if life had taught them that problems are best solved with force and effort. Others will succumb to their illness, allowing it to become the centre of their lives. They will identify themselves as patients, letting the illness get the upper hand. Pope Francis' method, with its additional specific applications, offers helpful directions for the sick, but also for healthy people so that they can take command of their lives as something that can be re-shaped. Leadership clearly starts with the self and one's own self-awareness. Patients assume leadership when they trust time more than space, unity more than conflict, realities more than ideas, and the whole more than a part. Leaders in the spirit of Pope Francis' method will occupy space from the middle and with respect for the purpose. They will search for unity in a conflict. They will re-ground ideas in reality. They will focus on the whole more than on any part. And they will "deal" with time!

What is helpful for an individual as a patient can also help physicians and nurses, as professionals in the healthcare system, to perform their leadership roles with responsibility and awareness.

I – 4: HOW HEALTHCARE PROFESSIONALS LEAD THE RELATIONSHIP WITH PATIENTS

Healthcare professionals and patients do not normally seek each other out – they are simply brought together by circumstances. Whether they like each other or not, they must communicate and cooperate. Physicians and caregivers are usually in a leadership role when they interact with patients, but outdated paternalistic attitudes are rightly no longer acceptable in the medical and caring professions. They are gradually being replaced by fairer forms of cooperation, based on an equitable relationship between mature adults. A manner of communication must be found that allows the healthcare professional to fulfil their leadership role competently, taking into account not only the patient's health issues but also their own and the patient's personalities. Now that patient autonomy has become a priority issue, a considerable amount of energy is expended on this tentative leadership concept. Although not all patients want their doctor to advise them on their autonomous decisions, physicians still need to evaluate each case individually and decide whether to simply assume leadership, in the sense of protective care-giving, or whether to obtain the patient's consent for each decision. In praxis, the professional expertise of physicians and caregivers means there are times when they have no option but to take on the leadership role and a large part of the responsibility for the patient. According to today's professional ethics, they may do this with the patient's assumed consent.

Especially when faced with an unfavourable prognosis, physicians as leaders must tackle a broad range of roles and tasks together with their patients and teams. To illustrate The Pope Francis Leadership Formula in a concrete case, I will use the example of a terminal illness. In this context, I will not focus primarily on doctor-patient communication (which will be discussed in the next chapter) or on the discourse among experts and the multi-disciplinary team, but rather on the intrapersonal professional and ethical considerations in the physician's or caregiver's *forum internum*. Faced with a confirmed, unfavourable prognosis for a patient, physicians will often have to wrestle internally with a number of professional dilemmas. They are required to disclose a patient's diagnosis and options in a way that preserves a patient's ability to decide about their treatment. Physicians and, to a certain degree, caregivers must deal with questions of how and when, where and with whom the treatment will be carried out. The purpose of the conversation with the patient is clear: the physician will truthfully explain the situation. Guided by their conscience, as a professional and a human being, they contemplate which path to take.

Reading the medical report for one more time, the physician recognises the patient's situation from long years of professional experience. The carcinoma — a pancreatic tumour — will spread quickly and unstoppably in the fifty-year-old patient's body. The patient has already been informed that it is a cancer diagnosis but he does not know the type of cancer, the probable turn the disease will take, or what treatment is available. The head physician's rounds will take place in a few minutes.

While considering the situation, the physician clearly must master the tension between **time** and **space**. In this case, "space" is the hard, indisputable fact of the diagnosis. The physician will have to work with "time" so that the patient will not be overwhelmed by the now unequivocal "space". Following the guidance of the formula, physicians must take time to learn about the patient's other spaces. When they are familiar with the patient's environment and family situation, their attitudes towards life and death, their history, and their dreams, then medical staff can begin to illuminate the new space together with the patient. The new space of the patient's illness won't disappear. But time can be shaped in a way that transforms the last space in the patient's life, so that they become master of it, rather than merely a dying person confined within the walls of a closed-in space. The art of dealing with time in a positive and healthy way is what characterises the bedside manner of experienced medical personnel and pastoral counsellors.

The right to receive truthful information and to be able to give informed consent does not morally contradict the preference for time over space. The question of how and when this space will be entered is more important than the fact of actually entering it. It must not lock the patient in or out. What matters is the patient's truth and not the truth of the space. It is important that the patient is not misled and, for instance, be given false hope that they can escape from this space. Between the two extremes of illuminating and denying the new space lies a vast grey area that permits an honest and helpful play with light and time. In a busy hospital with many physicians and caregivers, informing the patient is even more complicated, and harder on the patient, if the medical staff fail to take time to coordinate their approach to dealing with the unfavourable prognosis.

In such acute situations, the physician faces a serious prospect of professional and human conflict. Let us examine whether the second part of Pope Francis' Leadership Formula (**unity** is more important than **conflict**) can be helpful here. As long as the patient has not been fully informed, it will remain difficult to present the whole range of treatment options available. When the disease has progressed beyond a certain stage, there is nothing the surgeon, for instance, can do any more. If a patient still has many personal or professional affairs to deal with before they lose the ability, "dealing" with time must not be delayed too much. In making their own moral evaluations, physicians will have to make compromises with regard to colleagues, caregivers, the patient and his environment.

Every compromise necessarily resolves conflict in a certain way but there is a serious risk of losing sight of unity, i.e. the patient's welfare. Nevertheless, the formula would still suggest this approach. Applying it here does not mean making bad compromises just for the sake of unity. Any conflict should address legitimate concerns and become part of a new synthesis. At this point the physician can no longer avoid the case conference with his colleagues and the caregivers while considering how to deal with the prognosis. For the sake of unity, it is worthwhile spending more time "removing" the potential for conflict. Time invested in professional coordination will ultimately pay off, for the patient and the healthcare team.

To give priority to a conflict, even a conflict between authorities, will destroy unity (i.e. within the team and for the benefit of the patient) and will make it impossible to take other important needs into consideration for the moral evaluation. A physician or caregiver who adopts the weighting factors of leadership according to The Pope Francis Method will invest more time and energy in unity than in various conflicts. When dealing with the patient, this means giving priority to his overall and indivisible wellbeing. And when dealing with professional colleagues, it means investing time in collective solutions that take into account the important needs of different approaches, and therefore a solution, at a higher level (i.e. a different level to that of the protagonists). The logic of the formula does not sidestep the conflicts but rather uses them productively as a learning tool in the team and the whole hospital system so that it does not deteriorate into a soulless, unthinking bureaucracy.

Let us now turn to the formula's next area of tension — one that frequently afflicts physicians and caregivers, both individually and jointly as professionals: the relationship between **realities** and **ideas**. The impressive effectiveness of modern medicine owes much to the integration and skilful application of theories taken from many scientific fields, such as chemistry, physics, IT, technology, biology and neurology.

Medical theories continue to be developed on a daily basis, and the recourse to algorithms has become unavoidable in order to maintain an overview of the large amount of theoretical data. In addition, analyses and examinations of patients also provide enormous amounts of data. The "good practice" strategies of health insurance providers, along with competition in the health system and public access to data on the relative effectiveness of therapies, mean that physicians are under constant pressure to demonstrate that they are making decisions and acting in line with the most up-to-date scientific knowledge. Caregivers too must work to defined standards of care quality. This promotes the "idea" of good caregiving and good medicine in the health system, as well as in the eyes of the public.

As medical systems guided by standardised ideas become more complex, it becomes more difficult to introduce personal professional preferences. And it becomes increasingly difficult to appreciate the multifaceted reality of the entire patient, as opposed to the individual selected medical interventions in his body, or even merely his disease. The patient disappears behind the algorithms of the system, as do the physician and the nurses. They operate the systems professionally and apply them appropriately. Systems are becoming increasingly adept at integrating deviations in the patient and in their environments according to their underlying mastertheories. This creates an unrealistic enthusiasm for the application of artificial intelligence in medicine, based on a delusory understanding of its capabilities. A new concept – one that at first sight seems a positive step – demands our attention: personalised medicine.

The traditional therapeutic relationship between doctor and patient that has existed since the beginnings of medicine has been technologically extended. The so-called new personalised medicine is nothing more than the smart interaction of computers: machines containing patients' personal biological and genetic data along with their medical records are linked to other powerful computers that provide "the complete knowledge" of biology and genetics to create an "intelligent" system. As is the case with BCIs (brain-computer interfaces), the important element is the intelligent interface that provides the algorithm that enables the two computers to understand each other and exchange meaningful information. It is not my intent to criticise the introduction of technology and IT into medicine, but rather to point out the significance humans have assigned to this phenomenon through terminology. The new American term "personalised medicine" speaks volumes about the condition and dream of contemporary medicine and its progress.

Those of us who seek to challenge these powerfully eloquent ideas in a scientifically responsible manner can be grateful to Sir Karl Popper, the renowned philosopher of science who turned the logic of research on its head at the beginning of the 1930s. By giving priority to 'falsification' over 'verification' in attempting to prove or disprove scientific theories, Popper was, like Pope Francis, giving priority to realities, albeit using different words. The classic logic of 'verification' in sciences will repeatedly test even the most absurd theory against different elements of reality in order to eventually confirm it. It follows the logic of power, but not the logic of research.

Against this epistemological background, it is possible for physicians – as responsible scientists and researchers, as well as human beings – to calmly and honestly take command of the situation when dealing with diseases and patients. All they need to do is trust the patient's reality and the logic of 'falsification' more than general ideas and algorithms.

Doctors and nurses will ultimately benefit from opting to focus on the full reality of patients and their diseases and will thereby be able to reveal the true value of the person. From the perspective of dignity, the value of both the patient and their physicians and care-givers can be seen in their mutual engagement. In reality, so-called personalised medicine as a technical achievement has presented a vivid example of the value of humans over technical options and applications. A patient does not choose their physician as a medical technician but rather as a competent human being.

Bearing in mind that only humans are capable of dying with awareness, the bipolar tension of **realities** and **ideas** brings further drama to our case of a terminally ill patient and the deliberations of the medical team. If the "reality" of a patient, their disease, and especially their "time" are to take moral priority — according to the formula — then communication with the patient, and the treatments offered, must be adjusted to the patient's entire reality. This brings us to the next priority issue of the Leadership Method: the tension between the **whole** and the **part**. At first glance, one might think that this is about the tension we have just discussed. But on closer inspection you will see that reality itself consists of parts *and* of the whole. The fourth part of the formula therefore stands on its own, linking two specific sides of the octahedron.

In the face of human death, all issues present themselves in a different light. If terminally ill patients are regarded as walking, intelligent digestive systems, healthcare professionals will treat them differently than if they are regarded as individuals who want to shape themselves and their lives, and to think beyond death. Ultimately, in the face of death, technology and all the latest medical discoveries lose their glamour and persuasiveness. Even if these technologies had the potential to survive mankind, they would become obsolete without humans.

The drama of death, and even more so the drama of dying, has made man a unique being of nature. His creativity and ideas have enabled him to snatch back a fair amount of quality time from death. Mankind's technical extensions, coupled with human guile, have been helpful in evading certain natural processes. Before mankind subjects itself completely to technological developments that will soon be able to control themselves, it should once again be reminded of its original project of "man and society". This project held, and still holds, the claim to serve man's development as *homo sapiens sapiens* and was not intended to be the pre-stage of a higher developed species of *homo faber* that creates and possibly eliminates itself.

Death is an issue that concerns the person as a whole and the whole person. From this perspective, the parts lose their attraction and allure. Whether a person dies with a broken leg or an open wound is of secondary importance when compared to their death as a person. No good physician will lose sight of the interconnectedness within the whole. With this understanding, they will precisely assess which parts require attention and treat them as parts of the whole. This holistic approach requires physicians and caregivers to show courage and big-heartedness when dealing with the sick, and it requires patients to be courageous too. In the final analysis, it is not about a part that can be controlled; it is about a person with their own history, life, and ideas about the future. It is not easy, and not without risk, to get involved with a patient in this personal context. Here, healthcare workers are needed more as humans than as specialists, and much depends on how they integrate their personalities and competencies as professionals. What matters is not only how they deal with patients at the end of their lives but above all how they develop their own "self-portrait" or self-conception as professionals in the healthcare system. Their identities are formed in the day-to-day combination of their actions and reflection on those actions.

Good leaders — whether in the healthcare system or outside of it — are conscious of themselves and their jobs, thus confident in managing individual situations. They are self-aware, know their limitations and responsibilities, and deal with external influences in a professional way. In the case of healthcare professionals, The Pope Francis' Leadership Formula can help them to become and remain competent leaders in their relationship with patients.

I – 5: THE PHYSICIAN-PATIENT CONVERSATION AS A SPECIAL LEADERSHIP CHALLENGE

It is clear that both patient and physician can benefit enormously from the Leadership Formula. As leaders, each of them takes charge of their own self-determination, but how do we deal with the imbalance that exists due to the physician's superior professional knowledge and expertise regarding the patient's illness? This is an asymmetry that is common in various business areas. In order to balance the distinct advantage a competent professional has over a client, or patient, many professions have adopted their own code of ethics to guarantee that the advantages of expert knowledge or competence will not put the client at a disadvantage. Such a code of ethics – medical ethos probably being the oldest of them all – ensures, for example, that medical graduates can only go on to become licensed physicians when they have sworn to respect and abide by the codified commitments of their profession.

The current professional code of the German Medical Association[2] (2015), for example, has changed little with regard to a physician's duty towards patients. The obligation to provide information to patients remains a categorical imperative, and medical confidentiality remains a strict rule that can only be overridden by another rule or by the patients themselves. In this way, the doctor-patient conversation is well protected. Like the priest hearing a confession, the doctor promises confidentiality in order to promote trust[3]. There are often practical limitations to a "confessional situation", however, particularly in hospitals where physicians and nurses need to cooperate and communicate with each other about a case[4]. In this situation, professional codes dictate that a patient's consent must either have been obtained or can at least be presumed.

In contrast to the first two chapters (leadership in the sense of steering people and experts), this section deals with leadership in the context of thematic fields. This is probably the most common form of leadership experienced in today's world: What counts is the matter at hand and the direction to be taken on a particular issue.

If there is only one possible solution to an issue, then we do not require leadership, but merely expert knowledge. But when it comes to controversial issues, there is a need for much more than technical or factual knowledge. Indeed, important questions of ethics are

---

2) (Sample) Professional Code for Physicians Working in Germany in the Version of the Resolution of the 118th German Medical Assembly in Frankfurt am Main (Status: May 27th,.2015)
3) See the preamble of the Standard Professional Code, A.
4) Art. 9, 2,3,4.

usually at stake. Politics and the market economy are prominent witnesses of such battles for the right direction, which are usually fought in public. If an issue is initially resolved behind closed doors, increasingly often, public pressure will impose a second round on the secretive decision-makers. This may be prompted by the media or political groups and may sometimes even produce a different result to the first one. Think of how Volkswagen's emissions scandal was handled before and after the American and European public started to get involved. The same scrutiny is now given to medical issues. Class action initiatives (such as in North Rhine-Westphalia[5]), the introduction of patient representatives, and the proliferation of healthcare-related internet pages all reflect a growing interest in making the issue of illness a public one instead of an intimate discussion between physician and patient. And not a few medical scandals have shown that mistakes are just as much a part of daily life in medicine as they are in the lives of students, employees, politicians, and families.

Professional conversations with a patient are related to the current status and evaluation of their health and to the presumed developments, with their opportunities and risks. Again, **time** and **space** play a decisive role. A person's present state of health is a kind of spatial inventory; its development into the next space is a question of time. Physicians and patients are usually able to describe the health status rather well from their respective perspectives. This spatial approach to the subject of health, first of all, involves gaining a common understanding of the status quo. The words may differ but in the end they should express the same matter appropriately. Since describing health (or the disease) is a kind of "art",

---

5) See, for example, the i-Gel-Ärger-Internet site of the Consumer Assistance Center of North Rhine-Westphalia.

different emphases and nuances do not need to have a common denominator. Both parties only have to ensure that the same reality is being described.

This "spatial" description is complex enough by itself; but including the factor of time adds further difficulties when defining possible spaces for the future. According to The Pope Francis Formula, the physician would take the leadership role in this "context of time". Bringing his skills to bear, he is able to design a new space where the patient can feel at home within the limitations and options dictated by his illness.

Shaping time in this way, physicians must be like skilled architects who are able to draw the patient's future space as realistically and accurately as possible. At the same time, they are able to give patients the opportunity to contribute towards the design of their future spaces in terms of what is possible and realistic. The future perspective may be grey or dark; yet it presents horizons the patient can shape creatively. Good, experienced physicians know that what matters in such future-orientated conversations is less the upcoming surgical procedure or therapy than a concrete vision of the new physical-spatial home. The more concretely patients can envision the future — i.e., the time — the easier will be the medical decisions on the way there. Patients will gladly leave the technical decisions to physicians and nurses if they can be certain that all involved share the same goal for the treatment and are basing their activities on the same "plan". Then it does not matter all that much what is put where first, but rather that everyone agrees on an overall but flexible schedule. The fact that "time" is more important than "space" proves to be true here, too.

While the first part of the Formula, applied to the physician-patient conversation, suggests that the future design of the new or next phase of health must lead the conversation, the second one brings us to the **conflicts** and the **unity** that is endangered.

As long as the joint enterprise of working towards the patient's own health expectations and the planned outcomes continues, all conflicts that arise along the way must be addressed. The experienced physician will particularly address those conflicts that may be unpleasant for the patient or that have not yet been considered. How will he deal with his severely limited range of movement? How will he handle the fact that he will have to completely change his eating habits after a massive surgical intervention? It would be a mistake to assume that addressing future conflicts (the patient's current abilities and future abilities) would adversely affect his trust in, or even his willingness to consent to, a difficult intervention. On the contrary, the inner and bodily conflicts the patient will face should be used to paint a realistic picture of his new unity. If he focuses his energy on a realistic future of "unity" and "completeness", there is a chance to integrate the potential for conflict into the new picture. If the disease is a serious one, this new picture will not be the direct extension of the current or former state of health but rather a new synthesis. The more conflicts can be integrated physically and mentally into this new unity, the more readily their differences will be reconciled.

Dealing with the inner potential of conflicts does not provoke them but rather serves unity. Keeping conflicts under cover and not addressing them can, on the other hand, endanger unity more and continue to feed specific areas of conflict. The intelligence embedded in the Formula proves its worth here. Actively addressing conflicts in the interest of unity is valuable because every conflict contains material for a new and different future.

The third principle of the Formula takes us to the bipolar area of tension between **realities** and **ideas**. With this principle, Pope Francis brings movement into the area of tension by treating realities as more important than ideas. If the physician adheres to this leadership principle when talking to his patient, he will be able to credibly assure the patient that the common idea of a new "house of health" is important but that it needs to be adjusted to real progress or setbacks again and again. The patient will be better prepared to go along with an image of his future if he is aware of the fact that it is "only" an idea. On the other hand, he will find it harder to cope with if he feels that he surrendered all options for improvement or change when he gave his consent to his new health plan. This weighting between "realities" and "ideas" is helpful for the physician as well and reflects his scientific education in the sense of "falsification". Should any new facts or deviations from the planned treatment arise while realising the agreed strategy, they will be addressed.

In such a crisis conversation triggered by new facts, reality is paramount — rather than ideas about how to achieve the planned goal regardless of cost. Every experienced physician knows that certain events or circumstances will question the entire basis of a health intervention. The conversation must therefore be started anew based on the current facts. It never pays to lead a fictitious conversation from the perspective of a goal that has already become unachievable. In doing so, physicians would mislead the patient, discredit themselves as physicians, and create a conflict with professional ethics. Since the reality will always be stronger than the idea when it comes to concrete issues, it is advisable to face it and accept it as one's starting point; to do otherwise would be building castles in the air. In crisis conversations that are necessary along a path that has already been set, the physician will always keep the first part of the Leadership

Formula in mind and "deal" with time, without wasting it in the process.

The fourth part of the formula leads to the poles of the **whole** and **parts**. Diseases first affect one part of the body by affecting its functions. However, since our body is an interconnected, integrated system, even the smallest part affects our whole being. Any tiny localised pain reminds us distinctly that this correlation cannot be out-smarted. Therefore, the physician will always bring the patient's attention to their whole situation, as it is now and as it will be in the future. Directing a patient's attention away from their symptoms and concrete fears regarding any specific future deficiencies helps to give priority to the whole over its parts. In praxis, the physician and the patient know that any human being is a whole. But, when it comes to highly specialised medicine, both are especially at risk of focusing on one organ or function regardless of its context. The powerful corrective of the Leadership Formula is clearly also evident in the physician-patient conversation, and invites both to focus on the whole.

I – 6: THE LEADERSHIP FORMULA IN HOSPITAL MANAGEMENT

Today's hospitals have to manage the complex relationship between medical science and available resources. Good medicine requires good resources; and a well-equipped health system requires good doctors. The tension between the hospital as an economic enterprise and the hospital as a medical service run by doctors cannot be overstated, yet it represents the standard relationship between economics and medicine. Both deal with persistently scarce commodities. Neither medicine nor economics manages to achieve everything that is intended. That is why the management of hospitals cannot be left solely to either economists or medical experts.

In this chapter we examine whether Pope Francis' Leadership Formula can also promote wise and ethically responsible decisions in this area, stimulating action in a creative and methodically targeted way.

This issue, which dominates politics as much as it does the daily running of a hospital, concerns patients and physicians as well as administrative directors and health insurance providers. Governments hope that the invisible hand of the market will be the deciding factor in most cases. Health, however, is not a mere market-based product, but is rather a common good of the people. And what has actually happened is that the issue has been passed on to hospitals and delegated to physicians and their patients, without them being provided with the means to achieve an ethical resolution.

No reasonable person will question the fact that all resources are limited. This applies to money and to life itself. Both are finite. These two limited goods sometimes compete with each other, affecting us not only when our lives are restricted by disease or even death, but at other times of life as well. Take for example our dreams about our careers or leisure time that cannot be fulfilled because our resources are limited. As a result, a large number of ethical and political conflicts are caused by the way shortages are managed. Experience and morality teach us to live with shortages while simultaneously tackling the underlying causes. Unfortunately, as an issue of justice and rights, a shortage of goods is often of more concern than waste and abundance.

As a concrete example of how the Leadership Method can be applied in hospitals, let us consider the purchase of an expensive surgical instrument capable of carrying out delicate operations on a patient almost by itself, with minimum risk[6]. Such a robot is only used for very limited indications; and it should reduce the time the patient is hospitalised.

---

6) Robot-assisted prostate surgery may serve as an example.

The physicians and economists are not in agreement over whether such an acquisition makes sense – neither between the two groups of professionals, nor among themselves as individuals within each group. Yet a multi-disciplinary group needs to prepare an expert opinion for the decision-makers. Here again we may ask if, and to what extent, the Pope Francis Leadership Formula can be applied to these discussions.

In the **time-space balance**, "space" here incorporates various spaces. The robot itself is one such space. Its relationship to the operating theatre staff has to be clarified, because ultimately a physician will have to take responsibility for the surgery, performing it with an instrument that sometimes works independently but that he can "switch off" at any point. Taking into account the potential savings to be made in terms of time and money, the costs of the instrument represent another space factor that in turn is intimately connected to time. The "spaces" are well filled with difficult questions.

So how might the "time" factor be applied usefully in order to reach a decision if, for instance, it is itself an argument for acting fast to be one step ahead of competitors? The decision-making process is heavily burdened and requires intelligent action from the moderator of the multi-disciplinary group. If time becomes an obstacle to morally well-balanced decisions, it makes sense to postpone the arguments about time, scheduling the decision about the timing of the envisaged acquisition at the end of the process. The question of when the instrument is to be acquired must not be paramount either for the finance department or for the physicians, both of whom see the chance of a benefit. First and foremost, economical issues serve the whole, as does the medical perspective. From that viewpoint, we will now look at the fourth part of the Leadership Formula (the **whole** must have priority over the **part**), which thematically should be considered first.

Why does a hospital purchase such an instrument: because of its reputation, for reasons of medical quality and patient safety, the profit margin, the reputation of its top surgeons, to strategically position itself in a certain therapeutic field...? Only with an eye for this view and the whole picture will the jungle of questions and uncertainties thin out. And only if the participants in the discussion truly work towards a common answer, will any progress be made in the decision-finding process. The numerous and partly conflicting partial aspects of implementing the robot may be discussed in accordance with the second principle of the Formula. Since the purchase will only pay off if the instrument is used at least once per day while the actual number of patients would only justify about forty such applications per year, the question for the hospital as a whole system with physicians and patients is: Should this general hospital become a specialised clinic for particular diagnostics and a specific therapy?

If we assume that the hospital's catchment area potentially contains sufficient numbers of this type of patient, then the question is a strategic one. If the hospital decides to pursue it, it will gladly pay the price for this instrument and re-organise the facility so that it can re-position itself in its new role.

The answer to the question will be a different one if the main motive for the acquisition is to serve some patients and physicians through reducing the risk in this type of intervention. In that case, it is more a question of specialised surgery for a particular diagnosis. This would mainly be of benefit to a narrow group of patients and medical specialists. Here, the hospital could become a platform for communication and fundraising. From this perspective, the acquisition is no longer about the whole hospital but rather about an important part in a very specific area of surgery.

Depending on which of the scenarios outlined here applies, the internal and external conflicts will change. However, once the fundamental choice about the purpose of the acquisition has been made, a common picture of the "whole" arises and puts the different "parts" into a framework of references that should produce confidence about the proceedings. It is now clear that the hospital will either become a specialised facility or it will provide an important specialised form of treatment for a small number of people. From the perspective of public welfare, each individual is as important as the next one, but money invested in one medical speciality cannot be spent on another. For public medical facilities, the authorities will play a decisive part in the basic decision about the overall focus, thus ensuring that individual patients in a certain region have access to the same treatment options.

Thus, for the purpose of illustrating the Formula, let us limit the area of conflict to the internal hospital organisation and the internal competition between the different medical fields.

Before dealing with these conflicts, however, it would be useful to apply the third Formula, which assigns more weight to **realities** than to **ideas**. As we have already seen, an idea is considered to have been invalidated, if reality shows that it is not the case. The question of whether to purchase a highly specialised robot for a specific type of surgery raises further questions about practical experience in handling the instrument, training of future surgeons and the experience gained in actual operations at the hospital. Unreliable colleagues who shirk their responsibilities by putting their faith in future technologies will not be convincing. Reality is once again stronger than ideas.

If many days of training, as well as daily use of the machine, are required to maintain competency in using it, the option of a certain medical speciality will require a good deal of lobbying and funds in order to be convincing. Let us assume that the pro-robot lobby is persuasive because patients will be able to be released from hospital sooner and, therefore, other special medical fields will be able to treat more patients. They will have to convince their professional colleagues that surgery risks can be reduced dramatically and that they will be able to use the instrument properly even if the number of patients concerned may be low.

Fair distribution among the medical departments will be shifted by the (potential) acquisition. By giving evidence of their new competency supported by the robot, the lobbyists hope for more patients in the operating theatre who will need to stay in the hospital for fewer days. The colleagues can expect to have more patients in their medical field. Now the normal rule of supply and demand comes into play in a newly arranged field, in which everyone sees how they will benefit from it. After the decision to implement the idea, reality will catch up with everyone again.

Whatever the conflicts may be, what matters is that the participants solve them in a fair manner. Here, the second part of the Leadership Formula – that **unity** is more important than **conflict** – would apply. The discussions within the team of experts should be organised accordingly. The concerns behind conflicts, patient safety, number of patients, the balance among the medical specialities, etc. should be considered as much as unity. That is because the concerns behind the conflicts help to strengthen unity and to find new solutions at a higher level. A common fund for investments, that everyone contributes to and shares in, would represent a creative solution for all surgeons. The hospital could contribute to the fund and manage it.

In the end, the first part of the Formula, which deals with **time** and **space**, regains its operative meaning after agreement has been reached about the whole and the verifiable reality. As long as all parts battle with each other simultaneously, time is wasted and the stronger parties prevail. That is why, from the perspective of hospital management, it is wise to expose all aspects of the conflict and to publicly share it in a structured and transparent process among all colleagues concerned. Only when the purpose and the goal of acquiring a robot for specialised interventions are clear to everyone can "time" again be introduced as a balancing factor to the different mechanisms of distribution.

I – 7: USE AND BENEFITS OF THE FORMULA

In the previous four chapters we have seen how the Leadership Method has the potential to methodically introduce movement to a number of stagnant situations.

At first glance, the simplicity of the "Formula" is fascinating. By applying it, it is possible to grasp complex situations and translate them into a new language. This new language has the advantage of bringing everyone to the same level of understanding. Patients as well as physicians and nurses, social and pastoral workers have to leave their respective (technical) language behind and consciously decide to adopt this exciting formula of Pope Francis to frame their communication. The semantic and axiological frame of this language-game, with eight key words and four movable balances, is wide and deep enough to effectively shape a specific discourse able to encapsulate the phenomena of diseases, concepts of life, and the necessary decisions. Without getting lost in the multiplicity and versatility of language, the Formula provides an instrument for open discourse without prejudging the outcome. It is open for all of humanity and all visions of the future. This is its strength and at the same time its weakness.

The Formula shares the strong point of all formulas: it presents a complex reality in a manageable form. Labelling specific elements and putting them into a rule-based relation creates a method by which certain phenomena can be described and understood. At the same time, the intelligence behind the formula offers options to methodically influence the phenomenon being described. The Pope Francis Formula can be used to bring movement to a connected system that is rigid or in danger of becoming rigid. Altering the hanging balance of the structure, by giving priority to a certain side, triggers the motion - thus moving the whole structure.

Like any effective formula, the variables of the Leadership Formula can be filled with different intentions and goals. It is open to abuse, triggering motion where morally no motion is needed, or triggering motion that is morally reprehensible. Georg Simon Ohm surely did not envisage the electric chair when he developed his current-voltage formula. For moral evaluation, the use of an instrument (even a formula) depends on the purpose and intention of its application.

With regard to the application of the Formula in healthcare, I take it for granted that the purpose of any medical facility is the recovery, preservation, or improvement of a patient's health. In these circumstances the application of the formula would be morally correct. My second assumption refers to the intentions of those who apply it: They apply it with good intentions in order to support and accompany the patient to the best of their abilities.

In connection with his Formula, Pope Francis consistently speaks of multi-polarity, referring back to the polyhedron as an image. Of all the platonic solids, the octahedron with its eight triangular sides, best represents the axes and sides addressed in Pope Francis's Formula (see cover illustration or the website: www.the-franciscode.com). If you put the initial letters of the eight key terms (time, space, unity, conflict, realities, ideas, whole, part) on the octahedron, you create a playful eight-sided dice that can be used to trigger motion in difficult situations. To make the dice even more instructional and comprehensible you can put the more important terms (time, unity, realities, whole) in capital letters. This "leadership dice" can become a playful and reliable tool for those involved in decision-making in healthcare, starting with the patient and the physician. Putting this leadership dice on the table makes it clear that decisions are required. The dice thus becomes a symbol for situations that need to be unblocked.

Every time a patient or a physician asks "where do we go from here?", and whenever issues are no longer addressed or discussions stagnate, someone can put the leadership dice on the table and address the relevant areas of tension represented by the letters. For instance, how does the capital "R" for "realities" relate to the small "i" for existing ideas to make a certain therapy attractive for the patient? Whoever throws the leadership dice opens the discussion based on the Leadership Formula. They invite themselves and the other participants to bring motion into the situation. It does not matter whether the discussion is opened by addressing a conflict or a partial aspect that is emotionally paralysing. The leadership dice can be moved again and again so that all of its sides are discussed and the liberating weightiness of the capital letters becomes apparent.

This method is certainly not a universal remedy. It is merely an instrument that may be used with a warm heart and a cool head for the benefit of the patient. The discussion that has been opened about how the patient's health is developing will benefit all parties concerned and the hospital itself. The special leadership dice, together with a brochure for patients, could be issued to patients when they are admitted to the hospital. The medical personnel could learn in specific training sessions how to work creatively and skilfully with the dice. Over time it could even become the trademark of the hospital that uses it and therefore a feature of special ethical and spiritual quality! This leadership dice might render many other differences less significant. It is a vehicle for everybody, regardless of their moral preferences or so-called professional assumptions. The method helps many different people who are searching for a way out of stagnation, providing them with the impetus to move forward. Their diversity is their richness and shows the full potential of taking up the dice as a leadership method.

Of course, the Pope Francis Leadership Formula won't solve all problems automatically or by magic. Instead, it triggers processes that can contribute to personal or mutual moral development. To that extent it is a catalyst in the hands of the leader and not a supplementary algorithm for a lack of leadership! Pope Francis' way corresponds to a pilgrim's path with an open future. The decision to walk down that path requires courage and is the first step along the way. Everything starts with this first step!

PART TWO

LEADERSHIP TOWARDS AN OPEN FUTURE

II – 1: THE WAY FORWARD

The Leadership Method we encountered in Part One is also central to this second part, in which we take a closer look at the man behind this comprehensive formula and his path of leadership and reform within the Church and in the world. I will not only examine how Pope Francis describes his formula but also how he applies it in practice. In the encyclical *Lumen fidei*[7] (LF), which Pope Francis took on from Pope Benedict and then personally expanded, he explicitly set out two of the four principles, thus indicating at this early stage of his pontificate the enormous status they hold in his approach.

Aware that conflicts are inevitable, launching his encyclical on the feast day of the holy leaders Saints Peter

---

7) Pope Francis, Encyclical Letter *Lumen fidei* of the Supreme Pontiff Francis to the Bishops, Priests and Deacons, Consecrated Persons and the Lay Faithful on Faith, Vatican Press Online (Hereafter, "LF").

and Paul (who were themselves not free from tension) he succinctly declares that *"from a purely anthropological standpoint, unity is superior to conflict"*. Overcoming a conflict while integrating its concerns is *"to make it a link in a chain, as part of a progress towards unity"* (LF, 55). Later, he presents his perspective of an open future: *"Let us refuse to be robbed of hope, or to allow our hope to be dimmed by facile answers and solutions which block our progress, 'fragmenting' time and changing it into space. Space hardens progress, whereas time propels towards the future and encourages us to go forward in hope"* (LF, 57). His formula is dedicated to unity and the future. As a believer and a leader, he relies on the fact that life will always go on, and he is therefore not afraid of the question "Where do we go from here?" His open formula can be used by anyone who asks this question because they too know deep down that life will go on and that their personal and responsible contribution counts.

The simplest and most insightful definition of a leader is that he or she exerts real influence on the direction and impact of an organisation and that such leadership is experienced and understood both within and outside of the organisation. This certainly applies to Pope Francis, whom the global public has perceived as a leader since his election and papal inauguration in March 2013. But he is not a mere celebrity; he has taken a particular path and is leading the Catholic Church forward in the global world.

Let me now say a few words about the difference between managers, of whom there are many, and leaders, of whom there are few: Managers work in the system, and leaders work on the system. Managers take care of maintaining the systems and rules for which they are responsible; leaders set out to cut new pathways through the undergrowth. Leaders organise things in such a way that the purpose of their enterprise (in both senses of the word) will be successful. They take the initial and transitional chaos as their starting point and as the raw material for the next stage of the human endeavour.

Books and articles[8] have already been written about Pope Francis' leadership. Usually it is his modesty and ability to make decisions that is emphasised and presented as a kind of extraordinary trademark. At the same time, he also seems to embody a kind of "anti-leader", at least from the viewpoint of some commentators who confuse leadership with being aloof and all-powerful. I would like to show that this pope has a unique yet universal approach to leadership, an approach he explicitly discloses in his programmatic apostolic exhortation *"Evangelii gaudium"*[9] (EG)[10].

Pope Francis has a holistic approach to leadership. He makes use of the platonic solids of geometry to illustrate the interactions between his four principles. He speaks of the polyhedron in contrast to the sphere. He values a particular kind of polyphonic harmony instead of a beautiful uniformity that won't disturb. He likes harmony in form, sound and concepts. At this point we can already recognise that the model for this kind of harmony can be found in the structures of the universe that must be artfully developed on Earth. It follows, therefore, that the art of leadership can be acquired as a skill, based on competences.

---

8) See Chris Lowney, Pope Francis: Why He Leads the Way He Leads, 2013; Jeffrey Krames, Lead with Humility: 12 Leadership Lessons from Pope Francis, 2014.
9) Pope Francis, *Evangelii Gaudium* of the Holy Father Francis to the Bishops, Clergy, Consecrated Persons and the Lay Faithful on the Proclamation of the Gospel in Today's World. Vatican Press Online, 2013 (referred to hereafter as "EG").
10) Also see my contribution to the same subject: *Leadership in eine offene Zukunft. Die Papst-Franziskus-Formel*, which will be published in: Studia Teologiczno-Historyczne Śląska Opolskiego, Volume 36, in the fall of 2016.

Francis refers to the oldest universal science known to us: philosophy. In the times of Plato, philosophy systematically put into words the sum of knowledge available through science, experience and wisdom. It was the ultimate expression of science. It structured all knowledge into meaningful principles and translated them into tangible tools for mastering life itself. Through this understanding of an all-embracing "philosophy", and of a friendship with knowledge, Pope Francis builds his octahedron as a leadership formula. Like the early philosophers, he has understood that our words and terms have to become concrete actions in order to have an effect on reality. Then they may create either chaos or harmony. Pope Francis has opted for harmony in motion and has put mankind as leaders on the side of God who, according to the Bible, created the world from chaos. Just as God was clearly not daunted by the chaos of this world, so human leaders should not despair at chaos but rather organise it methodically and in a goal-orientated manner. That is the task of any leader.

In the following chapters I will depict the four principles contained in *Evangelii Gaudium* as an interconnected leadership system and show how it is applied intelligently in *Laudato si'*[11] and *Amoris Laetitia*[12]. In this context, I will restrict myself to Pope Francis's texts, although his Leadership Formula can also be seen in his actions, for example at the Synod of Bishops on the Family or in his reform of the Curia. Like the Church, his

---

11) Pope Francis, *Encyclical Letter Laudato si' of the Holy Father Francis on Care for Our Common Home*, Vatican Press Online (referred to hereafter as "LS").
12) Pope Francis, *Post-synodal Apostolic Exhortation Amoris Laetitia of the Holy Father Francis to Bishops, Priests and Deacons, Consecrated Persons, Christian Married Couples, and All the Lay Faithful on Love in the Family*, Vatican Press Online (referred to hereafter as "AL").

ethical leadership serves only one purpose, namely *"... to announce the good news about Jesus Christ"*[13]. And that already fulfils one condition of his formula: It presumes an explicit purpose!

---

13) Cardinal Bergoglio's speech was published by Cardinal Jaime Ortega with the consent of the Pope, as he confirms: a German translation can be found on the websites of Adveniat (presse/papst-franziskus/rede im Vorkonklave).

II – 2: THE POPE FRANCIS LEADERSHIP FORMULA

Pope Francis introduces his chapter on leadership[14] with the following words: *"Small yet strong in the love of God, like Saint Francis of Assisi, all of us, as Christians, are called to watch over and protect the fragile world in which we live, and all its peoples"* (EG, 216). We — meaning in this text all Christians[15] — are called to take on the deficiencies of the people and the world in which we live. In *Laudato si'* Francis uses the formula in such a way that it is offered to all human beings regardless of their affiliations. It deals with the common

---

14) The term "The Pope Francis Leadership Method/Formula" was coined by the author, not by Pope Francis. Pope Francis has repeatedly mentioned the four principles and applies them in his writings and work.

15) In *Laudato si'* the Pope addresses all people without discrimination and applies his formula of the *Evangelii Gaudium* quite naturally. Therefore one can assume that the formula is offered to everyone, not only Christians.

good and social peace, which, as the Pope clearly illustrates, are at risk. The task addressed with the Leadership Method is a political one. Leadership, after all, is by definition always political. It is about shaping and not about controlling. In order to become one human family, Francis writes in *Evangelii Gaudium* (220), an ongoing process is needed *"in which every new generation must take part: a slow and arduous effort calling for a desire for integration and a willingness to achieve this through the growth of a peaceful and multifaceted culture of encounter."*

He refers to the four classical principles of Catholic Social Teaching: human dignity, the common good, subsidiarity, and solidarity and then arranges his specific criteria around these four pillars. *"Progress in building a people in peace, justice and fraternity depends on four principles related to constant tensions present in every social reality,"* the Pope writes, formulating his vision for the Leadership Method as follows: *"In their light I would now like to set forth these four specific principles which can guide the development of life in society and the building of a people where differences are harmonized within a shared purpose. I do so out of the conviction that their application can be a genuine path to peace within each nation and in the entire world"* (EG, 221).

The leadership task that needs to be mastered is therefore the development of social coexistence in the sense of an organised world or, in other words: the reconciliation of differences in a joint endeavour.

The Pope Francis Leadership Formula:

Time is greater than space (EG 222)
Unity prevails over conflict (EG 226)
Realities are more important than ideas (EG 231)
The whole is greater than the part (EG 234)

II – 3: WHY TIME IS WORTH MORE THAN SPACE TO ETHICAL LEADERS

In the first principle of his Leadership Formula, Pope Francis refers to the bipolar tension between abundance and limitation. Humans experience abundance as something desirable, while they run up against a wall when it comes to limitation. Applied to time, this abundance stands for the horizon that stretches out in front of us, while limitation stands for a moment.

If, as leaders, we picture this bipolar tension in the light of Pope Francis's method, we can appreciate that his first principle will be: Time is more important than space. Addressing all leaders, at the global and local levels, he says: *"This principle enables us to work slowly but surely, without being obsessed with immediate results"* (EG, 223). He notes that sometimes *"spaces and power are preferred to time and processes"* (EG, 223) in social politics, and describes this as a sin (i.e.

wilful wrongdoing), saying: *"Giving priority to space means madly attempting to keep everything together in the present, trying to possess all the spaces of power and of self-assertion; it is to crystallize processes and presume to hold them back"* (EG, 223). He obviously prioritises processes, and condemns taking possession of spaces. He invites individuals and groups to opt for activities that promote and create new and inclusive dynamics. This should be done with determination and without timidity. Francis does not fear time, and he cites his blessed fellow Jesuit, Petrus Faber: *"Time is God's messenger"* (EG, 171).

Among Francis's actions, the Synod on the Family and the issues it considered are the most illustrative example of how he handles the principle. *Amoris Laetitia*, the published conclusion, states in paragraph 3: *"Since 'time is greater than space', I would make it clear that not all discussions of doctrinal, moral or pastoral issues need to be settled by interventions of the magisterium. Unity of teaching and practice is certainly necessary in the Church, but this does not preclude various ways of interpreting some aspects of that teaching or drawing certain consequences from it. This will always be the case as the Spirit guides us towards the entire truth (cf. Jn 16:13), until he leads us fully into the mystery of Christ and enables us to see all things as he does"* (AL 3). Pope Francis reminds us of his method at the very beginning of this document, which may well be his most explosive within the Church, and applies his first leadership principle to the Synod itself and its contents. Without hesitation, he exposes selective or assimilated formulations of truth to re-evaluation in the light of this principle. There is no eternal truth until Christ allows us to see everything from his perspective at the end of time. So Pope Francis's method is definitely not about "playing for time" (see his warning in AL 233) but rather about playing "with time", actively using it for the leader's tasks and the purpose of the organisation.

In practice, leaders have sovereignty over time, be it in an organisation, in politics, or in the economy. Those in power determine when it is time to talk about what, and possibly how as well. That is their right and even their duty if they want to use time as part of the process to achieve the purpose of their tasks. A standstill will occur – and space will take up time – whenever time is wasted and not used. Then space will become the coordinate of orientation. In space, time is likely to stand still. Wherever time prevails over space, it moves it along. Pope Francis expresses this almost poetically, and full of hope, in *Evangelii Gaudium*: *"Time governs spaces, illumines them and makes them links in a constantly expanding chain, with no possibility of return"* (EG 223). He explicitly illuminates his concern again in *Amoris Laetitia*, within the framework of the educational relationship[16].

This pope is aware of the reality of time. He understands that space is a reality and that it is narrow. He knows how to give time priority, because in the end it will dominate over all spaces. Any space that hopes to escape the passage of time intact will be eroded unless it is continuously readjusted to the parameters of the flow of time to which it is inevitably exposed. Time is more powerful than space. For that reason, smart leaders actively give priority to time and use it creatively.

Actively playing with time is often opposed to passively being overwhelmed by time. Here, too, the Pope reveals a deep understanding of the issues, reminding us of "*patientia*", patience. The principle helps us, he says, to *"endure difficult and adverse situations, or inevitable changes in our plans"* (EG, 223).

---

16) AL, 261

A wise leader therefore manages time actively and passively. It should be clear by now that it is leaders rather than their teams who bear the cost when playing with patience in the game of time. Here, the third leadership principle, which is linked to the other three, already shines through, namely, that reality has priority over ideas!

He concludes his considerations by citing Romano Guardini, whom he studied intensively during his so-called exile in Germany and Córdoba. He asks himself: *"Sometimes I wonder if there are people in today's world who are really concerned about generating processes of people-building, as opposed to obtaining immediate results which yield easy, quick short-term political gains but do not enhance human fullness"* (EG 224). Then he answers his question, quoting Guardini's The End of the Modern World[17]: *"The only measure for properly evaluating an age is to ask to what extent it fosters the development and attainment of a full and authentically meaningful human existence [...]"* (EG 224).

The Pope's first leadership principle is also applied in the social encyclical *Laudato si'* (LS). Here, too, it is fully and explicitly used within the framework of his discussion of political responsibility: *"The myopia of power politics delays the inclusion of a farsighted environmental agenda within the overall agenda of governments. Thus we forget that 'time is greater than space', that we are always more effective when we generate processes rather than holding on to positions of power. True statecraft is manifest when, in difficult times, we uphold high principles and think of the long-term common good"* (LS 178). With a view to the third criterion already mentioned, he talks about the greater danger of practical relativism[18]

---

17) *The End of the Modern World*, according to Note 182 in *Evangelii Gaudium*.
18) The allusion to theoretical or philosophical relativism is obvious. If former popes mainly focused on the theological-philosophical debate

"which is even more dangerous than doctrinal relativism" (LS 122; EG, 80).

The design of space and time by humanity is a highly moral task. Effective leaders can, with their powerful interventions, make a decisive impact on the space(s) and time(s) of others when designing and re-designing their world. People as actors, and especially leaders, participate in the process of creation. Human beings are not only creatures but also co-creators. They are not only subject to norms and conditions, they are also responsible for creating them.

In order to get things moving in the time-space tension, the question of priority must be addressed. Does space absorb time and — in an extreme case — make it stand still in a museum of stagnant time, or does time pull all existing spaces into the black hole of evanescence? The Pope, like any authentic leader, would not want either of the two extremes. He prefers to establish a rule of priority that brings things into motion. The Pope opts for time, knowing that space will always catch up with time, incarnating itself in space in order to become tangible in the moment. The courage to make decisions with determination comes through ever-flowing time[19], and keeping a hopeful eye on the still open future. If we fail to use this opportunity, as human beings we will see the death of our freedom and mission. Then we become cogs in the machine of other interests and the interests of others; we swim in the stream of time, through spaces we

---

about the truth of certain theories, Francis takes a different approach and points out that the questions and issues that matter in this world are first and foremost practical ones.

19) As Martin Heidegger had probably expressed himself. See Rüdiger Safranski, *Zeit. Was sie mit uns macht und was wir aus ihr machen.* Munich 2015, particularly Chapter 3 on the time of concern.

have not chosen and that pass by without touching us[20].

Moral decisions, and changes in the balance of the bipolar tension in favour of time, set the organisation in motion. Conflicts that have contributed to a stagnant balance become visible immediately. The next bipolar tension a leader will have to focus on concerns the coordinates of unity and conflict. Francis sets this tension in motion by opting for unity.

---

20) Francis describes the two extremes poetically: *"[...] In the first, people get caught up in an abstract, globalized universe, falling into step behind everyone else, admiring the glitter of other people's world[s], gaping and applauding at all the right times. At the other extreme, they turn into a museum of local folklore, a world apart, doomed to doing the same things over and over, and incapable of being challenged by novelty or appreciating the beauty which God bestows beyond their borders"* (EG, 234).

II – 4: WHY UNITY IS WORTH MORE THAN CONFLICT TO ETHICAL LEADERS

Any leader or ordinary person who has to manage a situation must employ targeted processes to overcome stagnation in space and time and bring them into movement, using the creativity and participation of all those concerned. Whether it is the development of the human family, an organisation, a policy or economic spaces, what matters is mutual trust.

In *Evangelii Gaudium*, Pope Francis describes three options for dealing with conflict: On the one hand, there is avoiding or ignoring the conflict, and on the other, there is allowing oneself to become bogged down or imprisoned in it. But he offers a third solution: *"It is the willingness to face conflict head on, to resolve it and to make it a link in the chain of a new process"* (EG, 227). This requires a strong personality and deep conviction: *"[…] unity prevails over conflict"* (EG,

228). The pope is convinced that the ambition to build unity urges us to find *"a solution which takes place on a higher plane and preserves what is valid and useful on both sides"* (EG, 228). He goes on to talk about a *"new and promising synthesis"* (EG, 230) and a *"reconciled diversity"* (EG, 230).

The underlying rationale for tackling conflicts in this productive manner can be found in his anthropology and theology. He unequivocally ascribes his option directly to the Gospel. He makes a fundamental moral decision affecting his intentions and actions. Others might choose the opposite course to that of Pope Francis in attempting to mitigate the tension in the axis of unity and conflict. The structure of time and the demands placed on leaders by their personal interpretations of faith can prompt them to resolve this tension in favour of conflict. Take the Greek philosopher Heraclitus, who died in 460 BC, and wrote: *"War is the father and king of all: some he has made gods, and some men, some slaves and some free."* This moral stance does not integrate existing differences but, influenced by those who are stronger, turns some into winners and others into losers. Though the losers will not lose their dignity as humans (as compared to gods) or as slaves (as compared to free citizens), they will nevertheless lose their freedom, and with it the space to shape their lives themselves.

This attitude is out of the question for the Pope and the Social Teaching of the Church. He clearly places his trust in the firm ground of unity and makes this principle a fundamental option. The essential equality of human beings prohibits slavery, or as Immanuel Kant, the philosopher from Königsberg, says: *"Always recognize that human individuals are ends, and do not use them as means to your* *end.*²¹" Our human rights culture has been built on that conviction and has been at risk time and time again. This primary anthropological decision lays the foundations for a special form of society and of living together.

According to Pope Francis, the fundamental preference for "unity over conflict" goes back to the history of salvation itself, as revealed to mankind in the life and death of Jesus of Nazareth. He starts with the individual: *"But if we look more closely at the biblical texts, we find that the locus of this reconciliation of differences is within ourselves, in our lives, ever threatened as they are by fragmentation and breakdown. If hearts are shattered in thousands of pieces, it is not easy to create authentic peace in society"* (EG, 229). In the same drama of the cross in which the world is torn apart, it comes together again in a new synthesis. And this drama of brokenness is first played out in the leader's own heart. Unhappy leaders cannot bring others together – they are too busy with themselves. They bring their internal conflicts into situations in which they should be mediators and figures of integration.

The second leadership principle of the Pope's formula links the first to the last two. If you look specifically at Chapter III of *Evangelii Gaudium*, you will find sparse mention of the second principle but looking at the whole text, you will find other sections where it is further elucidated. Unity does not mean uniformity, and it refers to the common task and not to individuals. Thus, in paragraph 117 we read that the unity of the Church is not threatened by its cultural diversity, if the latter is understood correctly. Contrary to the fact that *"we in the Church can sometimes fall into a needless hallowing of our own culture"*, this pope writes with equanimity that the Gospel has a trans-cultural content and therefore as a revelation

---

21) Immanuel Kant, *Groundwork of the Metaphysic of Morals; Immanuel Kant, Grundlegung der Metaphysik der Sitten, Akademie-Ausgabe Kant Werke IV, Walter de Gruyter 1968, p. 429.*

obviously cannot and will not be identified with any particular culture.

In the context of evangelisation, Pope Francis develops his positive understanding of reconciled differences further by noting: *"[...] but the Holy Spirit, who is the source of that diversity, can bring forth something good from all things"* (EG, 131). Accordingly, the source of differences is not people but rather the wealth of possibilities that reality holds, as in the many different approaches to tackling and solving a problem. Often there is not just one solution, but many diverse solutions. In unity, however, everyone must act together and allow themselves to become part of this togetherness. *"[...][the Holy Spirit] alone can raise up diversity, plurality and multiplicity while at the same time bringing about unity,"* he writes. *"When we, for our part, aspire to diversity, we become self-enclosed, exclusive and divisive; similarly, whenever we attempt to create unity on the basis of our human calculation, we end up imposing a monolithic uniformity"* (EG 131). In his handling of the opposition he faced regarding the Church's attitude to divorced persons who have remarried, this Pope has illustrated how to *"build communion amid disagreement"* (EG, 228). He faced all objections publically and humbly. In this way he endured conflict for the sake of unity and gently advanced the teaching of the Church in unity[22].

With his third leadership principle, Pope Francis takes the tension between realities and ideas into consideration to keep it alive for the sake of reality.

---

22) Eva-Maria Faber, Martin M. Lintner, "Theologische Entwicklungen in *Amoris Laetitia* hinsichtlich der Frage der wiederverheirateten Geschiedenen", German websites of theology and the Church (amorirs-laetitia.pdf).

II – 5: WHY REALITIES ARE WORTH MORE THAN IDEAS TO ETHICAL LEADERS

Any leader who wants to take action must be prepared to deal with conflict. They must ensure that all viewpoints are expressed, creating a synthesis that goes beyond the different points in dispute and attains a newly-arranged unity in diversity. Discussions about different viewpoints frequently focus more on ideas than on reality. Each theory is seen to be a particularly successful expression of the reality it describes. Nevertheless, like derivatives in the investments world that have no connection to real money and the real economy, there are also theories that exist for their own sake.

The initial cleansing process any leader has to carry out is to uncover reality again and reveal it for what it is. There can and should be debate — but it should support people in making progress towards unity and justice. It should not become bogged down in discussions about rigid theories and formulations, opinions and entrenched traditional practices, which will only lead to deadlock. To the leader, that means decisions should be based on facts and arguments and not on pure preconceptions and personal ideas, i.e., personal preferences. The bipolar tension Pope Francis wants to preserve is in a *"continuous dialogue"* (EG, 231) between realities and ideas. He judges certain ideas harshly: *"Realities are greater than ideas. This calls for rejecting the various means of masking reality: angelic forms of purity, dictatorships of relativism, empty rhetoric, objectives more ideal than real, brands of ahistorical fundamentalism, ethical systems bereft of kindness, intellectual discourse bereft of wisdom"* (EG, 231).

As he sees it, *"ideas – conceptual elaborations – are at the service of communication, understanding, and praxis"* (EG, 232). Personal and collective commitment is triggered by *"realities illuminated by reason"* (ibid.). The intended *"harmonious objectivity"* must be re-defined again and again in the course of time. Leadership can get lost in the heat of competing ideas without ever touching reality. The leaders concerned are separated from real operations, from the organisation or the corporation. They sit in their own worlds, entertaining themselves and others with their ideas about life, at the expense of reality.

The Pope writes ironically: *"We have politicians — and even religious leaders — who wonder why people do not understand and follow them, since their proposals are so clear and logical. Perhaps it is because they are stuck in the realm of pure ideas and end up reducing politics or faith to rhetoric. Others have left simplicity behind and have imported a rationality foreign to most people"* (EG 232).

In *Laudato si'* he refers to particularly dangerous and erroneous ideas that many people believe in despite the fact that they contradict with reality and their own experience: *"This has made it easy to accept the idea of infinite or unlimited growth, which proves so attractive to economists, financiers and experts in technology. It is based on the lie that there is an infinite supply of the earth's goods, and this leads to the planet being squeezed dry beyond every limit. It is the false notion that an infinite quantity of energy and resources are available, that it is possible to renew them quickly, and that the negative effects of the exploitation of the natural order can be easily absorbed"* (LS, 106). Accordingly, he quotes his third leadership principle in two significant sections of this encyclical (LS, 110; 201). *"In the concrete situation confronting us, there are a number of symptoms which point to what is wrong, such as environmental degradation, anxiety, a loss of the purpose of life and of community living. Once more we see that 'realities are more important than ideas' "* (LS 110).

In *Amoris Laetitia*, Pope Francis again shows explicitly how his various leadership principles are connected and work together: *"Don't get bogged down in your own limited ideas and opinions, but be prepared to change or expand them. The combination of two different ways of thinking can lead to a synthesis that enriches both. The unity that we seek is not uniformity but a 'unity in diversity' or 'reconciled diversity'. Fraternal communion is enriched by respect and appreciation for differences within an overall perspective that advances the common good"* (AL, 139).

This leadership principle, which at first glance seems so simple and insightful, is just as challenging as the two previous principles and the following one. It directs the leader to become involved in the action by facing reality. That is because hard reality will always prevail. Those who try to overlay it with theories and ideas will be rudely awakened. At that point it may be too late to correct the course. Our common home, as Francis calls the Earth in *Laudato si'*, is already burning while we discuss theories about melting glaciers and the greenhouse effect. In some branches of industry, hundreds of alarm signals have been overlooked and ignored because those in command do not want their self-fabricated world of ideas to be interrupted. Sooner or later reality will catch up with all of us. Therefore, it is better to face it in time and to work with it cooperatively and creatively with feasible ideas.

It almost seems as if the next and last leadership principle is merely another wording of the third one. "The whole is greater than the part", it states. However, since reality consists of parts and the whole, this is obviously not the case. Instead, the Pope refers to two other sides of his octahedron.

II – 6: WHY THE WHOLE IS WORTH MORE THAN THE PART TO ETHICAL LEADERS

Some leaders get lost in details. In colloquial language: they can't see the wood for the trees. That is one way of looking at the bipolar tension addressed here. Using the example of globalisation and localisation, Pope Francis says, *"Together, the two prevent us from falling into one of the two extremes"* (EG, 234). As is the case with the first three principles, it is not about balancing the tension but rather about creating motion and taking action, using the energy emerging from that tension. Pope Francis refers to rootedness, removing the abstract meaning of "global" in order to *"sink our roots deeper into the fertile soil."* Rather than being *"overly obsessed with limited and particular questions"*, we should *"constantly [...] broaden our horizon and see the greater good which will benefit us all"* (EG, 235).

He uses set theory to clarify his guiding principle and

reminds us that the whole is more than the sum of its parts. Then he goes on to explore the question of to what extent the part is a reflection of the entire mass it co-defines through its characteristics. The Gospel as a part is the sourdough that ferments the whole mass. It *"has an intrinsic principle of totality"* (EG, 237).

This pope accommodates the world community and all humans in a catholic way. Each part can contain everything, if it is part of the whole. And the whole can be reflected in very different parts. He states boldly: *"Even people who can be considered dubious on account of their errors have something to offer which must not be overlooked"* (EG, 236). By saying that, he looks with different eyes at more than one anathema from the past. He implies that traces of the truth might even be found in so-called mistakes, thus referring once again to the second leadership principle and its justification.

The tension must be sustained even though the whole has priority over the parts. The Pope concludes with the image of the polyhedron versus the perfect form of the sphere. He prefers the image of structures and developments that support themselves and that are permanently in motion — rather than that of the sphere, which rests in itself. In architecture, the term "tensegrity" (a *portmanteau* of "tension" and "integrity") was coined by Richard Buckminster Fuller to describe these structures. In today's view of anatomy or botany, creatures or growing plants are perceived as self-supporting structures. Francis uses the concepts of harmony and the polyhedron to illustrate his Leadership Method. The whole and the parts are mutually inter-dependent. If you want to get things moving, you will have to move everything in a tensegrity structure at the same time. That is why one should focus on the whole, i.e., the integrity of the self-developing structure. The gentle revolution heralded by Francis's

Leadership Formula moves everything and everyone simultaneously. He has confidence in the powers and intelligence of the human swarm. To this pope, God's people can be seen as a self-moving and organising swarm. No system of global governance can ever avoid placing its trust in the aggregate intelligence of self-aware citizens in a global society.

This wisdom is what characterises good leaders. They "deal" with time and, in a participative process, aim to creatively win everyone over for the intended purpose. Crucial conflicts have to be integrated or else the unity of the structure to be changed will collapse. This change does not happen in theory, but in reality. That is precisely why one has to be aware of the whole, which supports everything, and moves everything together at the same time. It cannot be predicted where and how the triggered movement towards another level will come to a (restful) stop again, since all powers are simultaneously challenged to interact and affect each other.

If leaders dare to tackle the system itself, leaving the comfort zone of their position of power in order to move a part of a balanced static organisation, they must influence everyone and everything; otherwise nothing will move, or everything will collapse. The insight provided by Pope Francis's Leadership Method shows why many leaders prefer to "wait and see", instead of tackling the system. Effective leadership is about all or nothing – and that even applies if everything remains stable, i.e., if nothing changes. This, too, is a question of all or nothing, of "to be or not to be". This pope was elected to set the system of the Church in motion and loosen its rigidity. He seems to reach many people, preparing them for the fact that unimaginable things may happen if everyone moves along.

That is why he addressed the *"diseases of the Curia"*[23] so harshly and offered his remedies in the following year.[24] As a "physician" preparing to perform painful surgical interventions, he hopes that compassion will lovingly move those with hardened hearts. His method follows the imperative of love and of the Good Samaritan. He does not want to leave anybody who is part of the whole at the roadside, for then he would betray himself as the leading shepherd. Like the Good Samaritan, however, he must rely on a stranger in an inn, who in return for payment will show pity and take the injured and down-trodden off his hands. Here, the whole global Church is challenged, not only as a hierarchy and structure, but as grass-root Christians and so-called lay faithful, as God's people on its pilgrimage into an open future.

---

23) Erny Gillen, *How a Pope Might Treat Curial Diseases. An Open Letter*, Luxembourg 2015. This public letter refers to the Christmas address to the Roman Curia of December 22nd, 2014.
24) See: Pope Francis, Address to the Roman Curia of December 21st, 2015.

CONCLUSION

All good leaders are aware of the role they play and the effect of their actions. They apply and implement their methods openly. They trust in an open future and leave it in the hands of God. They believe in the intelligence of the individuals in the organisation and use it to uncover the idiocy of the organisation[25], restoring its original purpose. If the purpose is clear — for instance, evangelisation in the case of the Church — they will continually find innovative approaches to bring the mission close to the people, enlisting the help of collaborators who actively and creatively participate in processes of transformation. Faith in the future is closely connected to faith in God who is One. Where faith represents the future it also keeps it open continuously for new approaches and endeavours.

---

25) See the works of Helmut Wilke.

As already mentioned, Francis's leadership principles depend on the question of whether a human enterprise knows its purpose and wants to serve it. As a society, we know the purpose of the economy, government and politics. If we as citizens, or believers, are prepared to accept our responsibility to be vigilant grass-roots leaders[26], the economy, government, and politics won't be able to resist the movement that can be triggered using the four tensions of the Leadership Formula. They will change according to their purposes, thus developing further into an open future.

There is great potential for the Pope Francis Leadership Method in our world, which he perceives as a *"sublime communion"* (LS, 89) in which everybody and everything are connected to each other because the One has created everything and everybody. The Pope calls us to live this deep togetherness in and with the whole of creation as a *"sublime fraternity"* (LS, 221). In this way he defines the purpose of political engagement, thereby enabling his Method to be used in responsibly setting our rigid worlds in motion and shaping them to serve the common good.

---

26) Niklas Luhmann, *Der neue Chef*, edited and epilogue by Jürgen Kaube, Berlin 2016.

ABOUT THE AUTHOR

Dr. Erny Gillen was a professor of theological ethics in Luxembourg for over twenty years. For ten of those years he also taught at the Catholic University of Applied Sciences in Freiburg, Germany, where he received the State Teaching Award of the Land of Baden-Württemberg in 2001. In the German-speaking countries he played a key role establishing Ethics Committees in Christian hospitals. In the field of medical ethics he taught and published prominent contributions discussing end of life decisions and praxis.

He practically applied his comprehensive expert knowledge to promote ethically underpinned morals while managing and developing Caritas in Luxembourg, Europe, and worldwide, as well as in other positions. Until May of 2015, he was the president of Caritas Europe (for two terms of office) and the first vice president of Caritas Internationalis in Rome. From 2011 to 2015 he took on responsibilities as vicar general within the archdiocese of

Luxembourg. Today he makes his expertise available as a consultant and keynote speaker for his company *Moral Factory* to a wide circle of interested people on an international level.

Erny Gillen has authored numerous publications, including a collection of lectures under the title *Wie Ethik Moral voranbringt* (*How Ethics Promote Morals*) (2006). *"How a Pope might treat curial diseases. An Open Letter"* to Pope Francis (2015) was written as his answer to the 2014 Christmas Address of Pope Francis to his Curia. It is published in four languages. *Neue Verhältnisse in Luxemburg – zwischen Staat und Religionsgemeinschaften"* (*New Relations in Luxembourg – Between the State and six religious communities*) (2015) illustrates the signed contracts resulting from negotiations between the government and six denominations. His contribution *Für eine Theologie der Moral und eine integrale Welt-Ethik. Wie Papst Franziskus Theologie und Ethik von innen heraus neu ausrichtet* (*For a Theology of Morals and Integral World Ethics. How Pope Francis Re-models Theology and Ethics from the Inside*)[27] was recently published.

---

27) In: Horizonte gegenwärtiger Ethik. Festschrift für Josef Schuster, SJ, Ed.: Paul Chummar Chittilappilly, Freiburg 2016, 268-279.

www.ingramcontent.com/pod-product-compliance
Lightning Source LLC
Chambersburg PA
CBHW030703190526
45164CB00004B/299

9 781536 843866